HEALING THE LIVER

A Comprehensive Guide To Treating Ischemia

Megan Williams

INTRODUCTION   **7**

UNDERSTANDING LIVER ISCHEMIA   **7**
DEFINITION AND CAUSES: 7
SYMPTOMS AND DIAGNOSIS   8
FATIGUE AND WEAKNESS   9
ENLARGED LIVER (HEPATOMEGALY)   9
DIAGNOSIS OF LIVER ISCHEMIA TYPICALLY INVOLVES A COMBINATION OF MEDICAL HISTORY REVIEW, PHYSICAL EXAMINATION, AND DIAGNOSTIC TESTS, INCLUDING   9
IMPORTANCE OF TIMELY TREATMENT   10
TIMELY INTERVENTIONS MAY INCLUDE: 10

CHAPTER ONE   **13**

LIFESTYLE CHANGES FOR LIVER HEALTH   **13**
DIET: FOODS TO INCLUDE AND AVOID   13
IMPORTANCE OF HYDRATION   15
EXERCISE AND PHYSICAL ACTIVITY RECOMMENDATIONS   16

CHAPTER TWO   **19**

HERBAL AND NUTRITIONAL SUPPLEMENTS   **19**
OVERVIEW OF HERBAL REMEDIES FOR LIVER HEALTH   19
ESSENTIAL NUTRIENTS FOR LIVER FUNCTION: 21
RECOMMENDED DOSAGES AND PRECAUTIONS   22

CHAPTER THREE   **25**

TRADITIONAL MEDICINE APPROACHES   **25**
ACUPUNCTURE AND ACUPRESSURE: 25
AYURVEDA AND LIVER HEALTH: 26
TRADITIONAL CHINESE MEDICINE PERSPECTIVES: 27

CHAPTER FOUR — 31

MODERN MEDICAL TREATMENTS — 31
MEDICATIONS FOR LIVER ISCHEMIA: — 31
INTERVENTIONAL RADIOLOGY PROCEDURES: — 32
SURGICAL OPTIONS AND CONSIDERATIONS: — 33

CHAPTER FIVE — 35

LIFESTYLE MANAGEMENT FOR LONG-TERM LIVER HEALTH — 35
STRESS MANAGEMENT TECHNIQUES: — 35
AVOIDING HARMFUL SUBSTANCES: — 36
IMPORTANCE OF REGULAR MEDICAL CHECK-UPS: — 37

CHAPTER SIX — 39

CASE STUDIES AND SUCCESS STORIES — 39
REAL-LIFE EXPERIENCES OF PATIENTS OVERCOMING LIVER ISCHEMIA: — 39
STRATEGIES THAT WORKED FOR DIFFERENT INDIVIDUALS: — 42

CHAPTER SEVEN — 45

PREVENTATIVE MEASURES — 45
EARLY DETECTION AND PREVENTION OF LIVER ISCHEMIA — 45
STRATEGIES FOR MAINTAINING LIVER HEALTH: — 46

CHAPTER EIGHT — 49

SUPPORT SYSTEMS AND RESOURCES — 49
SUPPORT GROUPS AND ONLINE COMMUNITIES — 49

CONCLUSION — 53

MOVING FORWARD: EMPOWERING YOURSELF FOR BETTER LIVER HEALTH   **53**

CREATING A PERSONALIZED PLAN FOR RECOVERY: 53

INTRODUCTION

Understanding Liver Ischemia

Definition and Causes:

Liver ischemia occurs when blood flow to the liver is restricted or reduced, leading to insufficient oxygen and nutrient supply to liver tissues. Ischemia can affect a specific area of the liver (focal ischemia) or the entire organ (global ischemia). Causes of liver ischemia include:

1. Hepatic Artery Occlusion: Blockage of the hepatic artery, which supplies oxygen-rich blood to the liver, can occur due to blood clots, atherosclerosis, or vasculitis.

2. Portal Vein Thrombosis: Clotting or obstruction in the portal vein, responsible for carrying nutrient-rich blood from the digestive organs to the liver, can lead to ischemia.

3. Surgical Procedures: Liver ischemia can occur as a complication of liver surgeries, such as liver resection or transplantation, due to temporary interruption of blood flow during the procedure.

4. Hypoperfusion: Conditions causing low blood pressure or shock can reduce blood flow to the liver, resulting in ischemia.

5. Liver Diseases: Conditions like cirrhosis, liver fibrosis, or liver cancer can compromise blood flow within the liver, increasing the risk of ischemia.

Understanding the underlying cause of liver ischemia is crucial for effective treatment and prevention of complications.

Symptoms and Diagnosis

Symptoms of liver ischemia can vary depending on the extent and duration of blood flow restriction. Common symptoms may include:

- Abdominal pain, especially in the upper right quadrant

- Nausea and vomiting

- Jaundice (yellowing of the skin and eyes)

Fatigue and weakness

Enlarged liver (hepatomegaly)

Diagnosis of liver ischemia typically involves a combination of medical history review, physical examination, and diagnostic tests, including

1. Imaging Studies: Techniques such as ultrasound, CT scan, or MRI can help visualize blood flow within the liver and detect any abnormalities or obstructions.

2. Liver Function Tests: Blood tests may reveal elevated liver enzymes or other markers of liver damage.

3. Angiography: Invasive procedures like hepatic angiography may be performed to directly visualize blood vessels in the liver and identify any blockages or abnormalities.

Early diagnosis of liver ischemia is essential to prevent further damage and initiate timely treatment.

Importance of Timely Treatment

Prompt treatment of liver ischemia is crucial to prevent irreversible liver damage and potential life-threatening complications such as liver failure.

Timely interventions may include:

1. Revascularization Procedures: Depending on the underlying cause, procedures like angioplasty, thrombolysis, or surgical revascularization may be performed to restore blood flow to the liver.

2. Medical Management: Medications to improve blood flow, reduce clot formation, or manage underlying conditions contributing to ischemia may be prescribed.

3. Supportive Care: In cases of severe ischemia or liver failure, supportive measures such as

intravenous fluids, nutritional support, and monitoring in an intensive care setting may be necessary.

Early recognition of symptoms, prompt medical evaluation, and initiation of appropriate treatment are essential for optimizing outcomes and preserving liver function in individuals with liver ischemia.

CHAPTER ONE

Lifestyle Changes for Liver Health

Diet: Foods to Include and Avoid

1. Include:

    - Fruits and vegetables: Rich in antioxidants and fiber, fruits and vegetables support liver health by aiding in detoxification and reducing inflammation.

    - Whole grains: Opt for whole grains like brown rice, quinoa, and oats, which provide complex carbohydrates and fiber without causing spikes in blood sugar levels.

    - Lean protein sources: Choose lean proteins such as poultry, fish, tofu, and legumes to reduce strain on the liver and support tissue repair.

- o Healthy fats: Incorporate sources of healthy fats such as avocados, nuts, seeds, and olive oil, which provide essential fatty acids and support liver function.

2. Avoid:

   - o Processed foods: Limit intake of processed foods high in refined sugars, unhealthy fats, and additives, as they can contribute to liver inflammation and damage.

   - o Sugary beverages: Reduce consumption of sugary sodas, juices, and energy drinks, as excessive sugar intake can lead to fatty liver disease and insulin resistance.

   - o High-sodium foods: Minimize intake of high-sodium foods like processed meats, canned soups, and salty snacks, as excessive sodium can contribute to fluid retention and liver complications.

- o Alcohol: Limit or avoid alcohol consumption, as it can cause liver inflammation, fatty liver disease, and liver cirrhosis.

Making dietary changes that prioritize whole, nutrient-dense foods and minimize processed and unhealthy options can significantly support liver health and function.

Importance of Hydration

Proper hydration is essential for liver health as it helps flush toxins from the body and supports optimal liver function. Adequate hydration also prevents dehydration, which can strain the liver and impair its ability to detoxify the body. Recommendations for staying hydrated include:

- Drink plenty of water throughout the day, aiming for at least 8-10 glasses daily.

- Limit intake of sugary and caffeinated beverages, as they can contribute to dehydration.

- Monitor urine color; pale yellow or clear urine indicates adequate hydration, while dark urine may signal dehydration.

Ensuring adequate hydration is a simple yet crucial aspect of maintaining overall liver health and supporting its detoxification processes.

Exercise and Physical Activity Recommendations

Regular exercise and physical activity play a vital role in promoting liver health by reducing liver fat, improving insulin sensitivity, and enhancing overall metabolic function. Recommendations for incorporating exercise into a liver-healthy lifestyle include:

- Aim for at least 150 minutes of moderate-intensity aerobic exercise or 75 minutes of vigorous-intensity exercise per week, as recommended by guidelines from health organizations.

- Include a combination of aerobic activities (e.g., walking, jogging, cycling) and strength training exercises (e.g., weightlifting, bodyweight exercises) to improve overall fitness and metabolic health.

- Stay active throughout the day by incorporating activities like walking, gardening, or taking the stairs whenever possible.

- Consult with a healthcare provider before starting a new exercise program, especially if you have underlying health conditions or concerns.

Regular physical activity not only supports liver health but also contributes to overall well-being and reduces the risk of chronic diseases such as obesity, diabetes, and cardiovascular disease.

CHAPTER TWO

Herbal and Nutritional Supplements

Overview of Herbal Remedies for Liver Health

1. Milk Thistle (Silybum marianum): One of the most well-known herbs for liver health, milk thistle contains active compounds like silymarin, which have antioxidant and anti-inflammatory properties. Milk thistle may help protect liver cells from damage and promote regeneration.

2. Turmeric (Curcuma longa): Curcumin, the active compound in turmeric, has potent antioxidant and anti-inflammatory effects. Studies suggest that turmeric may help reduce liver inflammation and improve liver function markers.

3. Dandelion (Taraxacum officinale): Dandelion root is traditionally used to support liver health and aid digestion. It may help stimulate bile production and

flow, promoting detoxification and liver function.

4. Artichoke (Cynara scolymus): Artichoke leaf extract contains compounds like cynarin and silymarin, which support liver health by increasing bile production and aiding digestion. It may also have antioxidant and anti-inflammatory effects.

5. Schisandra (Schisandra chinensis): Schisandra berries contain lignans and other compounds with hepatoprotective properties. Schisandra may help improve liver function and protect against liver damage caused by toxins.

While herbal remedies can offer potential benefits for liver health, it's essential to consult with a healthcare provider before starting any herbal supplement, especially if you have underlying health conditions or are taking medications.

Essential Nutrients for Liver Function:

1. Vitamin E: A potent antioxidant, vitamin E helps protect liver cells from oxidative damage and inflammation. Good food sources include nuts, seeds, vegetable oils, and leafy greens.

2. Vitamin C: Another powerful antioxidant, vitamin C supports liver health by scavenging free radicals and enhancing immune function. Citrus fruits, strawberries, bell peppers, and kiwi are excellent sources of vitamin C.

3. B vitamins: B vitamins, including B6, B12, and folate, play vital roles in liver metabolism and detoxification processes. Foods rich in B vitamins include whole grains, meat, fish, eggs, and leafy greens.

4. Omega-3 fatty acids: Found in fatty fish, flaxseeds, chia seeds, and walnuts, omega-3 fatty acids have anti-inflammatory properties and may help reduce liver

inflammation and improve lipid metabolism.

5. Selenium: Selenium is a trace mineral that acts as an antioxidant and supports liver detoxification pathways. Brazil nuts, seafood, organ meats, and whole grains are good dietary sources of selenium.

Ensuring adequate intake of these essential nutrients through a balanced diet is crucial for supporting liver function and overall health.

Recommended Dosages and Precautions

- Herbal supplement dosages can vary depending on factors such as the specific herb, its concentration, and individual health needs. It's important to follow the manufacturer's recommended dosage instructions or consult with a healthcare provider for personalized guidance.

- When choosing herbal supplements, opt for reputable brands that undergo quality testing and adhere to good manufacturing practices.

- Be aware of potential herb-drug interactions, especially if you are taking medications or have underlying health conditions. Always consult with a healthcare provider before adding herbal supplements to your regimen.

- Some individuals may be allergic to certain herbs or experience side effects such as gastrointestinal upset or allergic reactions. Discontinue use and seek medical attention if you experience any adverse reactions.

- Pregnant or breastfeeding women should exercise caution and consult with a healthcare provider before using herbal supplements, as their safety during pregnancy and lactation may not be established.

Incorporating herbal remedies and essential nutrients into a comprehensive approach to liver health can provide additional support for liver function and overall well-being. However, it's essential to approach herbal supplementation with caution and consult with a healthcare provider for personalized recommendations and guidance.

CHAPTER THREE

Traditional Medicine Approaches

Acupuncture and Acupressure:

1. Acupuncture: Acupuncture, a key component of traditional Chinese medicine (TCM), involves the insertion of thin needles into specific points on the body to stimulate energy flow (qi) and promote healing. In the context of liver health, acupuncture may help regulate liver function, improve blood flow, and alleviate symptoms associated with liver disorders such as pain and inflammation.

2. Acupressure: Acupressure involves applying pressure to specific acupuncture points using fingers, thumbs, or specialized tools. Similar to acupuncture, acupressure aims to balance the flow of energy in the body and promote health and well-being. Acupressure techniques targeting specific

points related to liver function may help alleviate symptoms and support liver health.

Ayurveda and Liver Health:

1. Liver Supportive Herbs: Ayurveda, the traditional healing system of India, offers a range of herbs and herbal formulations to support liver health. Herbs such as Kutki (Picrorhiza kurroa), Bhumi Amla (Phyllanthus niruri), and Punarnava (Boerhavia diffusa) are commonly used to detoxify the liver, improve digestion, and promote liver regeneration.

2. Diet and Lifestyle Recommendations: Ayurveda emphasizes the importance of maintaining a balanced lifestyle and dietary habits to support liver health. Recommendations may include consuming warm, cooked foods; avoiding processed and refined foods; and practicing regular detoxification techniques such as fasting or herbal cleansing.

3. Panchakarma Therapy: Panchakarma, a detoxification and rejuvenation therapy in Ayurveda, may be recommended for individuals with liver imbalances. Panchakarma treatments such as Virechana (therapeutic purgation) and Basti (medicated enema) aim to eliminate toxins from the body, restore balance, and rejuvenate liver function.

Traditional Chinese Medicine Perspectives:

1. Liver Qi Stagnation: In TCM, the liver is believed to govern the smooth flow of qi (vital energy) throughout the body. Liver qi stagnation, characterized by symptoms such as irritability, abdominal bloating, and menstrual irregularities, is a common pattern associated with liver imbalances. Acupuncture, herbal medicine, and lifestyle modifications are used to promote the smooth flow of liver qi and alleviate symptoms.

2. Herbal Formulations: TCM offers a variety of herbal formulations targeting liver health and addressing specific patterns of imbalance. Herbs such as Bupleurum (Chai Hu), Milk Thistle (Shui Fei Ji), and Rehmannia (Shu Di Huang) may be prescribed to tonify the liver, clear heat, and resolve dampness or stagnation.

3. Dietary Therapy: TCM dietary therapy emphasizes the importance of consuming foods that support liver health and balance the body's energy. Recommendations may include incorporating bitter and sour foods, reducing consumption of greasy or spicy foods, and maintaining regular meal times to support digestion and liver function.

Traditional medicine approaches such as acupuncture, Ayurveda, and Traditional Chinese Medicine offer holistic perspectives on liver health and provide a range of interventions to support liver function, promote balance, and alleviate symptoms associated with liver disorders. Integrating these modalities with conventional medical care may offer comprehensive support for individuals seeking to optimize their liver health and well-being.

CHAPTER FOUR

Modern Medical Treatments

Medications for Liver Ischemia:

1. Anticoagulants and Antiplatelet Agents: Medications such as heparin, warfarin, and antiplatelet drugs like aspirin or clopidogrel may be prescribed to prevent blood clots and reduce the risk of hepatic artery or portal vein thrombosis, which can lead to liver ischemia.

2. Vasodilators: Drugs that dilate blood vessels, such as nitroglycerin or nitrates, may be used to improve blood flow to the liver and alleviate symptoms of liver ischemia.

3. Thrombolytic Therapy: Thrombolytic drugs like tissue plasminogen activator (tPA) may be administered to dissolve blood clots and restore blood flow in cases of acute liver ischemia.

4. Pain Management Medications: Analgesic medications may be prescribed to manage abdominal pain and discomfort associated with liver ischemia.

Interventional Radiology Procedures:

1. Transarterial Embolization (TAE) or Chemoembolization (TACE): These minimally invasive procedures involve the injection of embolic agents or chemotherapy drugs directly into the hepatic artery to block blood flow to tumors or abnormal blood vessels feeding liver ischemia, thereby reducing ischemic damage or tumor growth.

2. Transjugular Intrahepatic Portosystemic Shunt (TIPS): TIPS is a procedure performed to alleviate portal hypertension and improve blood flow in patients with liver cirrhosis or portal vein thrombosis. A shunt is placed between the portal vein and hepatic vein to bypass the liver, reducing

pressure in the portal vein and improving blood flow.

3. Percutaneous Transhepatic Biliary Interventions: These procedures involve the insertion of a catheter into the liver to drain bile duct obstructions or perform interventions such as biliary stenting to alleviate symptoms and improve liver function in cases of biliary ischemia.

Surgical Options and Considerations:

1. Liver Resection: Surgical resection may be considered for localized liver ischemia or tumors affecting blood flow, with the goal of removing the affected portion of the liver while preserving healthy tissue.

2. Liver Transplantation: In cases of severe or irreversible liver ischemia, liver transplantation may be necessary to replace the damaged liver with a healthy donor liver and restore normal blood flow and function.

3. Acute portal vein thrombosis resulting in hepatic ischemia may be treated surgically with a portal vein thrombectomy, particularly in patients who have underlying clotting disorders or cancers.

4. Bypass Procedures: Surgical bypass procedures may be performed to reroute blood flow around blocked or narrowed blood vessels, restoring blood supply to the liver and alleviating symptoms of ischemia.

Modern medical treatments for liver ischemia aim to improve blood flow to the liver, alleviate symptoms, and prevent complications such as liver failure or tissue necrosis. The choice of treatment depends on the underlying cause, severity of ischemia, and individual patient factors, with a focus on optimizing outcomes and preserving liver function.

CHAPTER FIVE

Lifestyle Management for Long-Term Liver Health

Stress Management Techniques:

1. Mindfulness Meditation: Practicing mindfulness meditation can help reduce stress and promote relaxation by focusing attention on the present moment and cultivating awareness of thoughts and emotions.

2. Deep Breathing Exercises: Deep breathing exercises can trigger the body's relaxation response, reduce stress hormone levels, and foster feelings of calmness. Examples of these techniques are diaphragmatic breathing and the 4-7-8 technique.

3. Yoga and Tai Chi: These mind-body disciplines, which also include breathing exercises and meditation, combine physical postures with breathing exercises to lower

stress, increase flexibility, and improve general well-being.

4. Regular Exercise: Engaging in regular physical activity, such as walking, jogging, or cycling, can help reduce stress levels, boost mood-enhancing endorphins, and improve overall mental and emotional health.

Avoiding Harmful Substances:

1. Alcohol: Drink in moderation or abstain from it altogether as it can eventually cause fatty liver disease, liver cirrhosis, and liver inflammation.

2. Tobacco: Steer clear of tobacco smoke and products containing it, as these substances can harm liver cells and raise the risk of liver cancer and other liver diseases.

3. Illicit Drugs: Avoid the use of illicit drugs, as they can cause significant liver damage and increase the risk of liver-related complications such as hepatitis and liver failure.

4. Toxic Chemicals: Minimize exposure to toxic chemicals and environmental pollutants that can harm liver health, such as pesticides, industrial chemicals, and household cleaning products.

Importance of Regular Medical Check-ups:

1. Liver Function Tests: If liver function tests are routinely monitored, early indicators of liver damage or dysfunction can be identified. These tests may include blood tests to measure liver enzymes and other indicators of liver health.

2. Imaging Studies: Periodic imaging studies, such as ultrasound, CT scan, or MRI, may be recommended to evaluate liver structure and detect any abnormalities or signs of liver disease.

3. Screening for Liver Diseases: Individuals at risk for liver diseases, such as those with a history of viral hepatitis, alcohol abuse, or obesity, should undergo regular screenings

for conditions like hepatitis B, hepatitis C, fatty liver disease, and liver cancer.

4. Consultation with Healthcare Providers: Regular visits with healthcare providers, including primary care physicians, hepatologists, or gastroenterologists, can provide opportunities for health assessments, preventive care, and personalized recommendations for maintaining liver health.

By incorporating stress management techniques, avoiding harmful substances, and prioritizing regular medical check-ups, individuals can take proactive steps to support long-term liver health, reduce the risk of liver-related complications, and promote overall well-being.

CHAPTER SIX

Case Studies and Success Stories

Real-life Experiences of Patients Overcoming Liver Ischemia:

Case Study 1: Maria's Journey to Recovery

Maria, a 45-year-old woman, was diagnosed with liver ischemia due to portal vein thrombosis. She experienced symptoms such as abdominal pain, fatigue, and jaundice. After consulting with her healthcare team, Maria underwent a combination of medical treatments and lifestyle changes:

- Medications: Maria was prescribed anticoagulants to prevent blood clots and improve blood flow. She also received pain management medications to alleviate symptoms.

- Interventional Radiology: Maria underwent a transjugular intrahepatic portosystemic shunt (TIPS) procedure to relieve portal hypertension and improve liver blood flow.

- Lifestyle Changes: Maria adopted a liver-friendly diet rich in fruits, vegetables, and lean proteins. She practiced stress management techniques such as yoga and meditation and avoided alcohol and tobacco.

With the support of her healthcare team and dedication to her treatment plan, Maria experienced gradual improvement in her symptoms and liver function. Regular medical check-ups and monitoring helped ensure her continued progress and maintenance of liver health.

Case Study 2: David's Surgical Success

David, a 55-year-old man, was diagnosed with liver ischemia following liver resection surgery for liver cancer. Despite successful tumor removal, David developed ischemic complications due to temporary interruption of blood flow during the procedure. His treatment journey included:

- Surgical Options: David underwent a second surgery to address the ischemic damage and restore blood flow to the liver. Surgeons performed a bypass procedure to bypass blocked blood vessels and improve liver perfusion.

- Rehabilitation: Following surgery, David received post-operative care and rehabilitation to support recovery and optimize liver function. He participated in physical therapy to regain strength and mobility.

- Ongoing Monitoring: David continued to undergo regular medical check-ups and imaging studies to monitor liver function and assess for any signs of recurrence or complications.

Through surgical intervention, rehabilitation, and ongoing monitoring, David was able to overcome the challenges of liver ischemia and regain his health. His success story serves as an inspiration for others facing similar challenges.

Strategies That Worked for Different Individuals:

1. Early Intervention: Timely diagnosis and prompt initiation of appropriate treatment are crucial for improving outcomes in patients with liver ischemia.

2. Multidisciplinary Approach: A multidisciplinary team of healthcare providers, including hepatologists, interventional radiologists, surgeons, and nutritionists, can collaborate to develop individualized treatment plans tailored to each patient's needs.

3. Comprehensive Care: Integrating medical treatments with lifestyle modifications, such as dietary changes, stress management techniques, and avoidance of harmful substances, can provide holistic support for liver health and recovery.

4. Patient Education and Empowerment: Providing patients with information, resources, and support empowers them to

actively participate in their treatment journey and make informed decisions about their health.

By sharing real-life case studies and success stories, individuals can gain insights into effective strategies for managing liver ischemia and find hope and encouragement on their own path to recovery.

CHAPTER SEVEN

Preventative Measures

Early Detection and Prevention of Liver Ischemia

1. Regular Medical Check-ups: Schedule regular visits with your healthcare provider to monitor liver function and assess for any signs or risk factors for liver ischemia. Liver function tests and imaging studies can help detect early signs of liver damage or dysfunction.

2. Know the Risk Factors: Be aware of factors that increase the risk of liver ischemia, such as liver surgeries, portal vein thrombosis, liver diseases (e.g., cirrhosis, liver cancer), and conditions causing hypoperfusion (e.g., shock, low blood pressure).

3. Manage Underlying Conditions: Take steps to manage underlying conditions that may contribute to liver ischemia, such as

controlling blood pressure, managing diabetes, and treating liver diseases.

4. Medication Management: If you are taking medications that may increase the risk of blood clots or liver damage, work with your healthcare provider to monitor their effects and adjust your treatment plan as needed.

5. Healthy Lifestyle Habits: Adopt a healthy lifestyle that includes a balanced diet, regular exercise, stress management techniques, and avoidance of harmful substances such as alcohol and tobacco.

Strategies for Maintaining Liver Health:

1. Liver-Friendly Diet: Eat a balanced diet rich in fruits, vegetables, whole grains, lean proteins, and healthy fats. Limit consumption of processed foods, sugary beverages, and foods high in saturated and trans fats.

2. Stay Hydrated: Drink plenty of water throughout the day to support liver

function and promote detoxification. Limit
consumption of sugary and caffeinated
beverages.

3. Exercise Regularly: Engage in regular
   physical activity to improve overall health
   and reduce the risk of conditions such as
   obesity, diabetes, and fatty liver disease.
   Aim for at least 150 minutes of moderate-
   intensity exercise per week.

4. Maintain a Healthy Weight: Maintain a
   healthy weight through a combination of
   healthy eating and regular exercise. Excess
   weight, especially abdominal obesity, can
   increase the risk of fatty liver disease and
   liver complications.

5. Limit Alcohol Consumption: If you choose to
   drink alcohol, do so in moderation. For
   adults, this generally means up to one drink
   per day for women and up to two drinks per
   day for men.

6. Practice Safe Sex: Practice safe sex and
   avoid risky behaviors that may increase the

risk of sexually transmitted infections such as hepatitis B and hepatitis C, which can lead to liver disease.

7. Avoiding Toxins: Minimize exposure to environmental toxins and chemicals that can harm liver health, such as pesticides, industrial chemicals, and household cleaning products.

By adopting preventative measures and lifestyle strategies aimed at early detection and maintenance of liver health, individuals can reduce the risk of liver ischemia and promote overall well-being for the long term. Regular monitoring, healthy habits, and proactive management of risk factors are key to protecting liver health and preventing liver-related complications.

CHAPTER EIGHT

Support Systems and Resources

Support Groups and Online Communities

1. American Liver Foundation (ALF): The ALF provides resources, support groups, and educational materials for individuals affected by liver disease, including liver ischemia. Their website offers information on liver health, treatment options, and support services.

2. Liver Hope: Liver Hope is an online community and support network for individuals living with liver diseases, including liver ischemia. Members can connect with others facing similar challenges, share experiences, and access resources and information.

3. Inspire Liver Disorders Support Community: Inspire is an online health community where individuals affected by liver

disorders, caregivers, and healthcare professionals can connect, share information, and offer support. The liver disorders community includes discussions on liver ischemia and related topics.

4. Local Support Groups: Many local hospitals, medical centers, and community organizations offer support groups for individuals with liver diseases. These groups provide opportunities for networking, education, and emotional support.

Reliable Sources of Information and Assistance:

1. National Institutes of Health (NIH): The NIH offers comprehensive information on liver health, liver diseases, and related research initiatives. Their website provides educational resources, clinical trial listings, and links to other reputable sources of information.

2. Centers for Disease Control and Prevention (CDC): The CDC provides information and resources on liver diseases, including

prevention strategies, screening guidelines, and vaccination recommendations for hepatitis B and hepatitis C.

3. Mayo Clinic: Mayo Clinic's website offers reliable information on liver health, liver diseases, and treatment options. Their liver disease section includes articles, videos, and patient stories to help individuals understand and manage liver conditions.

4. Liver Specialists: Consult with hepatologists, gastroenterologists, or liver specialists for personalized guidance and medical advice. These healthcare professionals can assess your individual risk factors, provide recommendations for prevention and treatment, and coordinate care as needed.

5. Pharmaceutical Companies: Pharmaceutical companies that manufacture medications for liver diseases may offer patient assistance programs, educational materials, and support services for individuals using

their products. Check their websites or contact them directly for more information.

6. Patient Advocacy Organizations: Organizations such as the American Liver Foundation, Liver Hope, and the Hepatitis Foundation International advocate for individuals affected by liver diseases and provide resources, support, and assistance.

By accessing support groups, online communities, and reliable sources of information and assistance, individuals affected by liver ischemia can find valuable resources, connect with others facing similar challenges, and access the support they need to manage their condition and improve their quality of life.

CONCLUSION

Moving Forward: Empowering Yourself for Better Liver Health

Creating a Personalized Plan for Recovery:

1. Consult with Healthcare Providers: Work with your healthcare team, including hepatologists, nutritionists, and other specialists, to develop a personalized plan tailored to your specific needs and goals.

2. Identify Treatment Options: Explore various treatment options, including medications, lifestyle modifications, and supportive therapies, and collaborate with your healthcare providers to determine the most appropriate approach for managing your liver health.

3. Address Underlying Factors: Identify and address underlying factors contributing to liver ischemia, such as liver diseases, blood

clotting disorders, or lifestyle factors like alcohol consumption or obesity.

4. Incorporate Lifestyle Changes: Make lifestyle changes to support liver health, including adopting a liver-friendly diet, engaging in regular exercise, managing stress, and avoiding harmful substances.

Setting Realistic Goals and Monitoring Progress:

1. Set Achievable Goals: Establish realistic and achievable goals for improving your liver health, such as reducing inflammation, optimizing liver function, or managing symptoms associated with liver ischemia.

2. Break Goals into Actionable Steps: Break down larger goals into smaller, manageable steps to facilitate progress and maintain motivation. Focus on making gradual, sustainable changes over time.

3. Track Your Progress: Keep track of your progress by monitoring symptoms, tracking dietary and lifestyle habits, and recording

any changes in liver function or overall well-being.

4. Regular Check-ups and Monitoring: Schedule regular medical check-ups and follow-up appointments with your healthcare providers to assess progress, adjust treatment plans as needed, and address any concerns or challenges that arise.

Celebrating Achievements and Maintaining Motivation:

1. Acknowledge Progress: Celebrate achievements and milestones along your journey to better liver health, whether it's reaching a dietary goal, improving liver function, or adopting healthier habits.

2. Stay Positive: Maintain a positive mindset and focus on the progress you've made, rather than dwelling on setbacks or challenges. Recognize that small changes

add up over time and contribute to long-term success.

3. Seek Support: Lean on support systems, including family, friends, healthcare providers, and online communities, for encouragement, guidance, and motivation during difficult times.

4. Practice Self-care: Prioritize self-care activities that promote physical, emotional, and mental well-being, such as relaxation techniques, hobbies, and activities that bring joy and fulfillment.

By creating a personalized plan for recovery, setting realistic goals, monitoring progress, and maintaining motivation, you can empower yourself to take control of your liver health, optimize treatment outcomes, and improve your overall quality of life. Remember that every step forward, no matter how small, is a step in the right direction toward better liver health and well-being.